Six Pack

in

24 days

Complete Training Program for a well defined Six Pack

The information provided herein is stated to be truthful and consistent, in that any liability, in terms of inattention or otherwise, by any usage or abuse of any policies, processes, or directions contained within is the solitary and utter responsibility of the recipient reader. Under no circumstances will any legal responsibility or blame be held against the publisher for any reparation, damages, or monetary loss due to the information herein, either directly or indirectly.

Respective authors own all copyrights not held by the publisher.

The information herein is offered for informational purposes solely and is universal as so. The presentation of the information is without a contract or any type of guarantee assurance.

The trademarks that are used are without any consent, and the publication of the trademark is without permission or backing by the trademark owner. All trademarks and brands within this book are for clarifying purposes only and are the owned by the owners themselves, not affiliated with this document.

ISBN:
ISBN-13:

DEDICATION

Contents

Introduction

I want to thank and congratulate you for downloading the book, "**Six-Packs in 24 days**".

This book contains proven steps and strategies on how to make a well defined abdominal muscles, better known as six-packs, in 24 days.

Congratulations, you're about to burn a lot of fat in the shortest amount of time possible. You are also about to build a nice athletic body with a well-defined 6-pack.

The strategies that are in this guide and in the attached training charts will force your body to consume thousands of calories and burn pounds of fat while optimizing the hormonal environment and revitalizing metabolism.

Even if you do not have a well-established diet, the cumulative effect of these well-planned workouts will help you melt the stubborn fat in your abdomen, hips, and thigh etc. and build a truly defined and appealing body.

Have you ever seen pictures of guys on the internet who look absolutely ripped? They're real! And the truth is, they didn't start out their lives looking like that. Another truth is that any regular Joe, with the right method, technique and application can upgrade and get to look like the hot guys that a lot of girls crave for. And what's more? You can achieve all these without using even a smidgen of drug or any other muscle growing steroid.

Six pack abs have timeless appeal. Nowadays, almost every guy has a hidden desire or converting their flabby stomach into six pack abs.

But, it requires sheer devotion, time, and patience to obtain a six pack abs physique.

You primarily need to focus on two major tasks. The first one is losing fat and the second is building muscle mass. It is possible to achieve this through dieting and exercising consistently. It is possible to have the most toned and ripped abs if you are ready to work hard and sacrifice your favorite unhealthy food stuff.

All you need to do is get rid of a layer of fat which have covered your abs.

Just remember that once you get abs, you're not done yet. After getting your abs, you should have to work even harder to maintain it.

In the guide below you will learn more about planning the 24 days of training and how to execute different training styles.

Chapter 1

Structure of the Training Program

The 24 days of the well-defined six-pack training program are planned in the following way:

Day 1	Day 2	Day 3	Day 4	Day 5
Density 1 Cardio	Lactic acid 1 Conditioning	Power 1 Cardio	Metabolic 1 Conditioning	Active recovery 45
Day 6	**Day 7**	**Day 8**	**Day 9**	**Day 10**
Density 2 Cardio	Lactic acid 2 Conditioning	Power 2 Cardio	Metabolic 2 Conditioning	Active recovery 60
Day 11	**Day 12**	**Day 13**	**Day 14**	**Day 15**
Density 1 Cardio	Lactic acid 1 Conditioning	Power 1 Cardio	Metabolic 1 Conditioning	Active recovery 75
Day 16	**Day 17**	**Day 18**	**Day 19**	**Day 20**
Density 2	Lactic acid 2 Conditioning	Power 2 Cardio	Metabolic 2 Conditioning	Active recovery 90
Day 21	**Day 22**	**Day 23**	**Day 24**	
Density 1 Cardio	Lactic acid 1 Conditioning	Power 1 Cardio	Metabolic 1 Conditioning	

This is the recommended structure of the program —the one that burns as much fat as possible and defines your six packs as well in just 24 days.

Overlapping these days of training on weekdays does not matter for program results. Every day you start the program will vary from one week to the next one.

If you have to make a day of rest just keep going from where you left off.

Chapter 2

The Training Styles

The training program for Six packs in 24 days is based on 7 different types of training to attack fat in as many possible ways without losing muscle.

The basis of the program, which you should concentrate your effort on, consists of the following training styles:

1- Power Training

Muscle strength training is the essential component of a smart weight loss diet plan.

The more strength and muscle mass you have, the more exercise you will make will require more from your body and you will be able to burn more fat.

Obviously, in this short, 24-day period, you cannot really build up your strength and lose weight at the same time.

However, boosting strength throughout this program will be very useful simply because it will induce the body's need to keep all types of muscle fibers.

In addition, to burn as much fat within this defined period, the strength training you use will not be a classic one: breaks are shorter, some exercises are grouped in supersets, and to facilitate the use of heavier weights along the training, the number of series is not predefined.

This means you will not go with the idea of doing 5 series of 5 repetitions, but you will know that you have to make a total of 25 repetitions using a weight of 5 maximum reps.

Even though, mathematically, it seems the same, in reality, things are different:

For example, let's say that during your normal workouts you gradually increase your weight and realized that to "chest BENCH PRESS" you can make 5 reps with 80 kg, but at 6 you have difficulty pushing up.

In this case, you may consider that 5 maximum repeats for this exercise are 80 kg.

If you were to make a warm up (normal warm up), and then try the 5 series of 5 repetitions using this weight of 80 kg, you most certainly have not succeeded.

You simply cannot work so much with a weight that is too much for you. It means that, after 2 or a maximum of 3 series, you will have to reduce it to continue.

That's why the solution that I recommend for strength training in this program is to not think about the number of series, better on the number of repetitions.

Power training involves heavy weight, high sets, and low reps ranging from 4–5 sets of 3 reps, 5–6 sets of 1–2 reps, or up to 7–8 sets of a single rep.

The benefits of power training are immense. Apart from the fact that being powerful will make you badass, it is a critical trait that allows athletes to jump high, hit hard, sprint fast, and makes them exciting to watch. Training for power will help you to build and strengthen your fast-twitch muscle fibers and your nervous system so that they have the capacity to generate explosive movements that are characteristic of the top athletes.

As a beginner or a low-intermediate lifter, you can make gains in many areas at once through *periodization* i.e. (a planned structure of your training regime used to dictate reaching certain goals at certain times) But, if you're a high-intermediate to advanced lifter looking to become more powerful, just concentrate on that alone or you'll risk under-developing in many other areas instead of making real gains in one. There are lots of methods to use for power training, so, it is advisable to also do additional research and find the one that is most in line with your specific power target.

2- Density Training

The density of a workout refers to the amount of work you do in a certain amount of time and is given the amount of exercise related to the time you are doing.

Workouts that have as the main method of progression density escalation burn a lot of calories and increase your ability to work and endurance to strength, being so good for both fat burning and muscle development.

As we say, the density of a workout is the amount of work reported in time of execution. So, in order to increase density, either increase the amount of work, or decrease the time you do this work, or a combination of these two.

The method you will rely on during the next 24 days of workout is focused on increasing the amount of work at the same time, Further progression is not only from one workout to another, but also from one series to another.

Let's say you have to do the next exercise:

Squats-maximum reps in 45 seconds

Bench Press (chest) – maximum reps in 30 seconds

Bent-Over Dumbbell Row – maximum reps in 30 seconds

For the first series you choose a weight that you think you could do about 10 to 15 reps:

    1a) Squats-12 reps with 55 kg

    1b)Bench Press (chest)-15 reps with 40 kg

1c) Bent over Dumbbell Row-13 reps with 15 kg (with one hand)

Then to force your workout density to increase, you will increase both the weight and the number of repetitions you do during that time:

1a) Squats-14 reps with 60 kg

1b) Bench Press (chest)-18 reps with 45 kg

1c) Bent over Dumbbell Row-15 reps with 17,5 kg (with one hand)

Even if at first sight it seems impossible to increase the weight and the number of repetitions, in this case, everything is possible.

The first series, even if it is heavy, will make you consume a significant amount of calories, will prepare your nervous system for the challenge of the second set, in which you will surpass your previous performance and stimulate the burning of a larger amount of body fat.

However, before you hit the gym, I have a few tips to take with you:

A. Start Slow and Easy:

If within the first set, you "blow your load", you will most definitely pay with the rest of your session. What you should do to avoid having a poor session is to recognize and accept the fact that number of reps you'll hit per set will reduce as you get to the end of your work time.

Whichever rep goal you choose, you should make sure to start with a weight that will allow you to hit that number for at least the first three sets. If, on your first set, you're barely able to grind out that last rep, reconsider your starting weight.

B. *Combine exercises that focus on muscle groups that are not in direct competition:*

Although they're short, density workouts can be extremely intense. Because of that, you'll want to get the most out of each exercise. To do so, and still be able to be to about your activities the next day, all you have to do is pair antagonist muscle groups instead of synergists.

However, what you want to achieve is a great pair of biceps then, pairing chin-ups and biceps curls might not be the best option. Instead, you should begin to alternate between chin-ups and dips which would allow you to go hard on both exercises without exhaustion and without one hindering the other.

As you go from one session to another, you'll find that you're beginning to take on more reps than before, gradually, with the same weight. Once you get a 20% increase in reps compared to where you initially started, you should increase your weight. The principles are few, but the methods are many.

3- Training of Lactic Acid

The primary reason you want to stimulate a large amount of lactic acid is the production of the "growth hormone" that occurs with it.

In addition, the training methods you use to get as much lactic acid are excellent for emptying glycogen stores and burning fats because they are very challenging, demanding much from the body.

Since lactic acid is produced especially by placing muscles under tension for a long time, all exercises in this training will be done at a slow pace of 3-4 seconds on the positive side and controlled in rest.

One thing you will surely notice is the difficulty of this style of training.

That is why you will have to reduce the weight normally used in exercises and use a lower one with 20-25%.

Lactic Acid Training causes your muscles to fail due to the lower cellular pH (the acid lowers pH, which is the acid-base balance in the blood. When it gets too low, your muscles are unable to contract effectively). Not being able to contract effectively protects the muscles from excessive breakdown, which is critical to preserving muscle mass under reduced-calorie conditions, i.e. dieting.

Lactic Acid Training also burns quite a lot of calories during the session itself. This is because of the very short rest periods and high volume of work. This, in turn, keeps your heart rate in an aerobic conditioning zone even during the rest, further increasing the benefits of the training. Increased Growth Hormone levels also increase the use of fat for energy during recovery after intense exercise. This means your body will be burning fat in order to help you recover from your training! As well, high-rep Lactic Acid Training trains the Type 1 muscle fibers (endurance-oriented), developing and multiplying the cellular energy furnaces known as mitochondria, which rely greatly on fats to supply energy to your cells. This means your body will become more productive at burning fat even while at rest. The high volume of the training you will be doing will also help to stimulate Growth Hormone production. Higher training volume has been shown to produce a better Growth Hormone response than lower-volume training. The high-rep qualities of the training helps to develop circulation in the muscles by increasing the number of capillaries (tiny blood vessels) feeding the muscles. More circulation means more nutrients which means easier muscle growth down the line!

4- Metabolic Conditioner

The metabolic conditioning routines are extremely effective, managing to cause the burning of a large amount of body fat relative to the time invested, without any of the disadvantages of cardio.

The best thing about Metabolic Conditioning is the fact that the high levels of intensity will help you burn more calories during and after your workout. The exercises, which include your whole body and compound movements, will help you lose fat and gain muscle more quickly and more efficiently than cardio or strength training alone.

With MetCon, you get more strength, power and endurance because, not only are you targeting every one of your energy pathways in one workout, you're also conditioning your body on every level.

Another benefit of MetCon is the high level of fitness that comes with it. If you can workout at that high level of intensity, then you can be rest assured that in every other thing you do each day, you'll easily pull through without feeling without qualms.

People enjoy MetCon workouts because they have so much variety. You're not slogging on a treadmill for 45 minutes to nowhere. You're doing a variety of exercises that will keep both your mind and body engaged

Metabolic conditioning is short and sweet. You have to work very hard, of course, but the payoff is you only have to do it for 10 or 30 minutes.

The simplest and most effective Method of Metabolic Conditioning that I recommend is called Training in high intensity ranges.

It is based on short intervals of intense effort, interleaved with rest periods or medium effort.

For the intensive effort part you can use:

Sprints

Climbing the stairs

Bicycle

Skip the rope

For this training method, choosing the way you work is yours, because, you and only you can see how much energy you have after completing your basic training.

5 Metabolic Resistance Training

Metabolic Resistance training is probably the most effective and often used method of burning body fat.

The main reason they rank first in the top of the weightlifting training for fat burn is the EPOC phenomenon (Excess Post Exercise Oxygen Consumption). It is the metabolic disorder that keeps your metabolism high hours after training.

Although, the other types of training in this program incorporate the concept of circuits to a certain extent, Metabolic resistance training focuses on this direction using two large circuits and one smaller to maximize the effect of EPOC and burn as much fat.

The primary exercises used in MRT work multiple large muscle groups at once. This stimulates the release of testosterone, which is a naturally produced steroid hormone that is essential for the muscle-building process.

Strenuous workouts increase your body's sensitivity to insulin—the storage hormone—which helps shuttle nutrients into muscles after a workout, when they need to repair and recover. Increased insulin sensitivity means that your body needs to release less insulin to do its job, which makes you a more efficient fat burner.

Combining heavy compound movements with minimal rest effectively stimulates the release of natural growth hormone, which builds muscle, burns fat and helps you recover faster for the next workout. And don't neglect your sleep. Large amounts of growth hormone are released at night.

For starters, throw out your old method of weight training. Performing one exercise at a time for three sets of eight to 12 repetitions simply does not have a place in MRT.

The best strategy is to alternate between large upper- and lower-body movements, so that one muscle group can rest while you work the opposing muscles. Strive to take the minimum amount of rest between sets that will leave you with enough energy to maintain your exercise technique.

Finally, the exercises I have chosen are more than just composing, moving the body in a more complex way in all its plans.

6- Cardio

The term "cardio" normally refers to medium to long-term exercise movements. The truth is that it is neither effective nor healthy. Furthermore, it cannot build you a really attractive body by itself.

And this is proven by studies and the experiences of thousands of people.

However, when you want to burn as much fat as possible in a really short time, a cardio session next to a properly planned workout will help you burn more calories.

Before you begin with cardio, there are some few tips you will have to keep in mind:

1) Plan your workout out ahead of time: you should know and have an idea about exactly what you want to do even before you step foot on the treadmill, track, or street.

2) Be strategic with your timing: If you always end up skipping out on your cardio, then you should do it when you first get to the gym or during the days when you're "off work". Cardio isn't about when you do it, the most important thing about cardio is that you don't skip your routine.

3) Focus on the task at hand: If you have a magazine or book you're reading and desperately want to finish up while you're working out, please stop it. You will not achieve your goal this way. No one's ever achieved

their desired level of fitness while reading and at the same time doing their cardio. You have to concentrate on one task, in essence, you have to choose which is more important at that moment. Your workout or the book you want to finish reading?

4) Complete your thorough warmup: Doing a dynamic warmup will increase your mobility, it will also decrease your chance of injury and prepare your body's systems in advance for the exercise. If you skip your pre-cardio warmup, you are bound to get hurt.

5) Avoid steady-state cardio: Unless you're training for a long-distance race, avoid staying at the same pace for an extended period of time on the treadmill. Vary your degrees of intensity which is also known as HIIT (high-intensity interval training) and you will witness an increase in your metabolism in a way that constant workout on the treadmill won't.

6) Work in sprints: Incorporate sprints into either your normal run or as a part of their own workout session. Sprints increases your metabolism and can assist with building muscles in your legs.

7) Mix in bodyweight exercises: Try mixing in bodyweight exercises between your runs. This will break up a "boring session" and add a strength-building component to your workout.

8) Fight the urge to stop: Ignore that voice in your head that tells you to slow down, take a break, or just flat-out quit. Fitness is a discipline. Learn to embrace the work.

9) Take breaks: Bring your heart rate right back down. This will improve your recovery process and progressively slow the body down after an intense session.

10) Keep track of your routines and PRs: the same way you keep a workout log of how much weight you lift is how you should also keep track of how far you went and the tempo you used to get there. The Numbers are always an accurate indicator of the work done. Documenting your progress will keep you in tune with what works and what doesn't.

11) Champion consistency: One great cardio session has never gotten anybody anywhere. Get into a routine and stick with it. Develop a process from warmup to cool down.

Finally, I should add that there are classical disadvantages of cardio such as sabotaging the hormonal environment, catabolism of muscle mass and slowing metabolism will be minimal.

The key is to keep a moderate intensity.

7- Active recovery

You cannot train intensely every day without negative repercussions. Therefore, in order to burn more calories without requiring additional muscle mass and nervous system, the best solution is to add walking sessions to the slow pace.

This seemingly trivial activity may even speed up your recovery after intense training, compared to the state of the chair.

Active recovery, may have several distinct advantages. Some believe that active recovery workouts help prime your body's metabolic pathways of recovery.

Some believe active recovery is idealized, and claim that less intense exercise simply does not add to training stress. It is argued that light workouts do not stimulate an added benefit to recovery; they are simply easy enough that they do not stop the body from recovering as it would.

Regardless of the mechanism many have seen benefits to including active recovery in their fitness plans. For some, the psychological benefits of active recovery are apparent. Many people feel better when they exercise daily. Movement has the capability to elevate mood among other positive attributes.

A huge point to consider is that some people find it easier to adhere to their diets on days they are active.

Lastly, it is important to note that daily movement provides the opportunity to burn a few extra calories, thus potentially aiding in losing fat.

8- Nutritional advice

Nutrition is extremely important when you want to lose weight. Even more if you want to do it in a healthy and lasting way.

If you currently have a well-rounded nutrition, you know how many calories you should eat, touch your protein needs, and avoid various toxins and less healthy foods-Congratulations

If you do not have the habit of eating healthy, or following certain principles, but just eating how it feels normal and how you have been accustomed throughout your life, now is not the time to start a diet, or to start making major changes in your daily nutrition.

The training plan you will follow will be very taxing and will help you burn body fat even if your nutrition is not up and running.

The last thing you want to do is to start bothering yourself in the evening or to get an important source of calories from your nutrition and torment your body even more. If you do this, you will be totally exhausted, you will feel tired and unwell every day and will be unable to train yourself enough to get impressive results.

If you still feel the need to do something nutritionally, start with the following tips:

- Replace every gram of sugar, juice, coffee and ice cream, biscuits or other sweets that you regularly consume with one gram of meat, eggs or whey protein.

- Consume mostly carbohydrates after training. If so far you eat a slice of bread at every meal, you now try to eat the whole bread only after training.

- Replace margarine or other fat-containing products with hydrogenated natural fat sources such as butter, almonds, avocados, olive oil, etc.

- Avoid frying in oil, but replace some of the oil lost with olive oil added to salads.

9- The proper training

9.1- Density training 1

Each circuit (groups 1,2 and 3) is executed twice. Choose a weight with which you can perform 10-15 repetitions and try to make as many repetitions as possible during the allocated time.

After completing the first series, increase the weight by 10 15% and try to do more repetitions than the first time. Rest for 20-30 seconds between exercises and maximum 2 minutes between circuits.

Note the number of repetitions and weights used to overcome them in the future.

	Exercise	Time
1	Dumbbell Reverse Lunge	45 seconds
	Dumbbell Romanian Deadlift	45 seconds
	Kettlebell Lateral Lunge	45 seconds
	Weighted Crunch	60 seconds
	Pause 2 minutes	
2	Chest Rotation Incline Press (Dumbbells)	45 seconds
	Bent-Over Dumbbell Row	45 seconds
	Deep Barbell Back Squat	60 seconds
	Dumbbell Biceps Curl	30 seconds
	Pause 2 minutes	
3	Arnold Press - Shoulder Exercise	45 seconds
	Oblique Twist "Wood Chopper	30 sec one side

9.1- Training for Lactic Acid 1

Exercise the exercise groups (1,2 and 3) below in circuit mode. Follow the specified tempo and try to move the highest weights for the recommended number of repetitions. Execute dynamic interruptions only once after completing the previous circuit.

	Exercise	Tempo on the positive side	Reps
1	bulgarian squats with dumbbells	3	15
	Bent over lateral raises	3	12
	Dumbbell Push Press	4	12
	Dynamic interruption Burpee 10 reps as fast as possible Side Plank 25 seconds each side		
2	Reverse Lat Pulldown	3	12
	Back Extension	4	15
	Dip Exercise	3	12
	push-ups as many as you can in 30 seconds		
3	Hanging Knee Lifts	3	12
	Goblet Squat	4	15

9.3- Strength training 1

Execute exercises using such heavy weight that it does not allow you to do over the number of reps specified in MR (maximum repeats).

If you have not estimated the correct weight and you can do more reps than the MR number, increases weight by 20% and continue on.

Continue with the maximum weight found until you reach the total number of reps . Rest your 60 seconds to exercises performed by single and 30 seconds on circuits (2 and 4)

	Exercise	Weight	Reps
1	Front Squat	8-10 MR	35
2	Bench Press	3-5 MR	25
	Dumbbell Row	3-5 MR	25/Hand
Dynamic interruption : Jumping Lunge Exercise make as many you can in 45 seconds			
3	Deadlift	5-7 MR	35
4	PUSH PRESS	9-12 MR	40
	Pull Up	6-8 MR	30
Dynamic interruption : push ups make as many you can in 45 seconds			

9.4- Metabolic Training 1

Execute each exercise group 3 times with a break of 15 seconds between exercises and 60 seconds between circuits. After the last series of the last exercise in the first circuit rest for a maximum of 3 minutes and continue with circuit 2. Take note of your performance in every series and try to overcome it every time.

	Exercise	Reps
1	Dumbbell Step Ups	10 each foot
	One-Arm Dumbbell Bench Press	10 each hand
	Alternating Dumbbell Row	10 each hand
	Single Leg Romanian Deadlift	10 each foot
	Plank	Maximum time
	pause 3 minutes	
2	Dumbbell Romanian Deadlift	12
	Pull Up	12
	Thruster	12
	Back Extension	12
	Push Up	maximum time

9.5- Density training 2

Each Circuit (Groups 1, 2, and 3) execute 2 times. choose a weight with which you can perform 10 15 reps and try to make as many repetitions as possible during the allocated time. After completing the first series, increase the weight by 10-15% and try to do more reps than the first series.

Rest at no more than 20 30 seconds between exercises and up to 2 minutes between circuits. Note the number of repetitions and weights used to be able to surpass them in the future.

	Exercise	Time
	Goblet Squat	45
1	Pull Up	30
	Dips	30
	Oblique Twist "Wood Chopper	30/Side
	pause 2 minutes	
	Bulgarian Split Squat	30/Side
2	Dumbbell Shoulder Press	45
	Dumbbell Hammer Curl	60
	Dumbbell Flys	45
	pause 2 minutes	
3	Decline Push-Up	45
	Crunches	60

9.6- Training for Lactic Acid 2

Execute exercise groups (1,2 and 3) below in circuit mode. Respect the specified tempo and try to move as high weights as possible to the recommended repeat rate. Rest as little as you can 5 10 seconds between exercises and 30 to 60 seconds between the circuits. Execute dynamic interruptions only once after completing the previous circuit. Note the number of reps made and the weight used in each series.

	Exercise	Tempo/positive side	Reps
1	Front Squat	6	15
	Flat Bench Dumbbell Flys	3	12
	Dumbbell Pullovers	3	12
Dynamic interruption push ups as many as you can 30 seconds			
2	Dumbbell Romanian Deadlift	3	15
	Barbell Bent-Over Row	3	12
	Arnold Press	3	12
Dynamic interruption **Mountain Climber as many as you can 30 seconds**			
3	Bulgarian Split Squat	4	12/leg
	Hanging Leg-Lift	3	10

9.7- Strength training 2

Execute exercises using such heavy weight that it does not allow you to do over the number of reps specified in MR (maximum repeats).

If you have not estimated the correct weight and you can do more reps than the MR number, increases weight by 10 - 20% and continue on.

Continue with the maximum weight found until you reach the total number of reps. Rest your 60 seconds to exercises performed by single and 30 seconds on circuits (2 and 4).

	Exercise	Weight	Reps
1	Bent Over Barbell Row	4-6 MR	35
2	Barbell Bench Press	3-5 MR	30
	Bent-Over Dumbbell Row	3-5 MR	30/Hand
Dynamic interruption Burpee as many you can in45 sec,			
3	Front Squat	8-10 MR	35
4	PUSH PRESS	9-12 MR	40
	Pull Up	6-8 MR	25
Dynamic interruption Jumping Lunge Exercise make as many you can in 45 seconds			

9.8- Metabolic Training 2

Execute each group of exercises 3 times with a break of 15 seconds between exercises and 60 seconds between circuits. After the last series of the last exercise in the first circuit rest for a maximum of 3 minutes and continue with circuit 2. Take note of your performance in every series and try to overcome it every time.

Exercise	Reps
Skater Squats	8 each foot
1 Leg Push-ups	8 each side
Bulgarian Split Squat	8 each foot
Dumbbell Row	8 each hand
Side Plank	30 sec /side
Pause 3 minutes	
Thruster one hand	10 each hand
Pull Up	10
Lunges	10 each foot
Dumbbell Side Lateral Raise	10
Knee Raises	10

Bonus!

wouldn't be nice to know when Amazon's top kindle books go on Free Promotion ? well now it's your chance!!

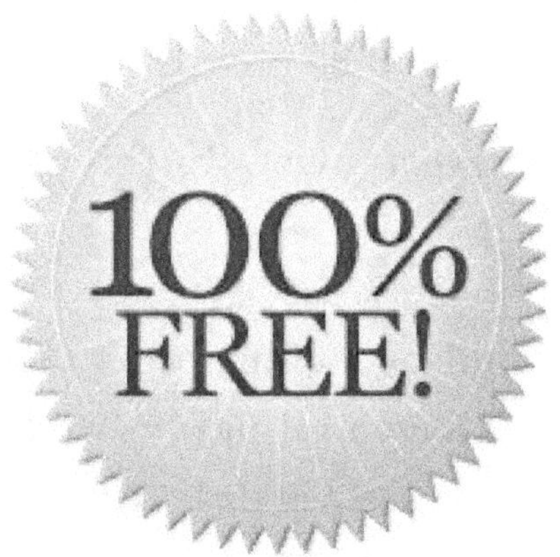

Click here for Instant Access!!!!

Simply as a thank you for downloading this book ,I would like to give you full Access to an exclusive services that will email you when Amazon's top Kindle books go on free promotion ,If you are someone who is interested in saving a lot of money ,than simply click the link for instant Access !!

Conclusion

Thank you again for downloading this book!

I hope this book was able to help you .

Finally, if you enjoyed this book, then I'd like to ask you for a favor, would you be kind enough to leave a review for this book on Amazon? It'd be greatly appreciated!

Click here to leave a review for this book on Amazon!

Check Out My Other Books

Below you'll find some of my other popular books that are popular on Amazon and Kindle as well. Simply click on the links below to check them out. Alternatively, you can visit my author page on Amazon to see other work done by me.

www.ingramcontent.com/pod-product-compliance
Lightning Source LLC
Chambersburg PA
CBHW060822260726
48660CB00003B/1052